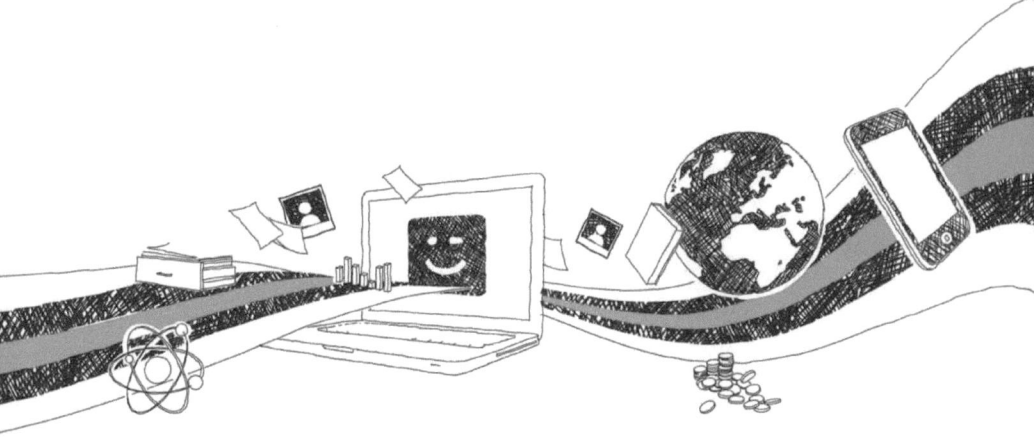
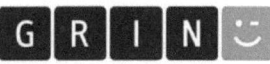

Leonard Kabongo

# Clinical and Epidemiological Analysis for HIV-exposed Infants in a Low Resource Setting: Evidence-based of PMTCT Interventions

GRIN Publishing

**Bibliographic information published by the German National Library:**

The German National Library lists this publication in the National Bibliography;
detailed bibliographic data are available on the Internet at http://dnb.dnb.de .

**Imprint:**

Copyright © 2011 GRIN Verlag, Open Publishing GmbH
Print and binding: Books on Demand GmbH, Norderstedt Germany
ISBN: 978-3-640-90941-4

**This book at GRIN:**

http://www.grin.com/en/e-book/171530/clinical-and-epidemiological-analysis-for-
hiv-exposed-infants-in-a-low

**GRIN - Your knowledge has value**

Since its foundation in 1998, GRIN has specialized in publishing academic texts by students, college teachers and other academics as e-book and printed book. The website www.grin.com is an ideal platform for presenting term papers, final papers, scientific essays, dissertations and specialist books.

**Visit us on the internet:**

http://www.grin.com/

http://www.facebook.com/grincom

http://www.twitter.com/grin_com

LEONARD KABONGO TSHIBASU

INTRODUCTION TO CLINICAL EPIDEMIOLOGY

CLINICAL AND EPIDEMIOLOGICAL ANALYSIS OF HIV-EXPOSED INFANT IN A LOW RESSOURCE SETTING: EVIDENCE BASED OF PMTCT INTERVENTIONS.

ATLANTIC INTERNATIONAL UNIVERSITY

HONOLULU   HAWAII

JANUARY 2011

# TABLE OF CONTENTS

**ABBREVIATIONS**

AIDS: Acquired Immune-deficiency Syndrome

ANC: Antenatal clinic

ARTIs: Acute Respiratory Tract Infections

AZT: Zidovudine

CFR: case fatality rate

CI: Confidence interval

DNA: Deoxyribonucleic acid

HAART: Highly Active Antiretroviral Therapy

HIV: Human Immunodeficiency Virus

HR: Hazard ratio

IMCI: Integrated Management of Child Illness

MTCT: Maternal To Child Transmission

OR: odds ratio

PCR: Polymerase Chain Reaction

PMTCT: Protection of Mother to Child Transmission

RNA: Rubonucleic acid

RR: Relative Risk

SdNVP: single dose Nevirapine

UCI: Universal Child Immunization

VCT: voluntary Counselling and Testing

WHO: world health organization

3TC: lamivudine

# Introduction

a. Definitions:

Clinical epidemiology is a fundamental epidemiologic approach based on the application of epidemiologic principles and methods in clinical setting. It's a basic science of medicine (Bonita R, Beaglehole R, Kjellestrom, 2008).Its approach considers using epidemiologic principles and methods to make clinical decisions and to measure outcome of disease.[3]

Mostly, clinicians deal with individuals whilst epidemiologists deal with communities. Thus, the concept of clinical epidemiology seems to be contradictory with its application. However, the current increase of knowledge in clinical medicine and pharmacology, the curiosity of knowing the validity of laboratory tests, the quest of a final and correct diagnosis and the necessity of cost-effective and efficient therapies, made the role of epidemiology more and more imperative. In this era called "pharmacoepidemiology", researchers focus on the advantages and disadvantage of drugs, hence their effects. This let Kenneth Rothman, 2002 to say: "outcomes research marries epidemiologic methods with clinical decision theory to determine which therapeutic approaches are the most cost-effective". [10]

This approach has lead to the concept of evidence –based medicine where sufficient proof are available to support a medical theory in disease management and promotion of various guidelines useful in clinical setting.Nonetheless, more medical and non medical conditions are still undiagnosed, under- diagnosed or wrongly diagnosed. As a consequence, extra, less cost-effective and unnecessary treatments are being prescribed. In this scenario, would the key to evidence- based medicine lie on diagnosis processes which are opaque to quantification and analysis, or on the deep-rooted knowledge of disease natural history, its transmission chain and physiopathology, or on the accuracy of diagnostic tests which have different level of interpretations according to their sensitivity or specificity? Or on prevention inputs to control the disease outcomes? These bottlenecks are generally and globally faced by clinicians whereas apply epidemiologic principles and fundamentals to research in clinical setting. This is not a question of controversy; Once understood and correctly applied, epidemiologic methods will raise a flow of evidences to audit the daily practice and make clinical decisions to amend or support existing therapeutic or management theories based on the findings.Again, implementation of new evidence-based innovations should be tested and completed.Recently, as discussing global health issues, Madon T et al ,2007 expressed concerns over most of discovered evidence-based theories that are not consistently tested or completed. [12]

In this research work, basic epidemiology principles and methods are applied to study the implication of PMTCT (Protection of Mother to Child Transmission of HIV) interventions in neonate populations born from HIV positive mothers in a low resource setting in Zambia.

b.Background:

In Zambia, roughly 80,000 infants are born annually from HIV infected mothers and are at risk of contracting the disease. An average of 20,000 are born with HIV each year (40%).The rate of vertical transmission varies from 15-25% in non-breastfeeding infants and double in breastfeeding ones. (Ministry of Health, National Protocol Guidelines, 2010). [14]

Over 9.2million children aged<5 years die every year in developing countries. (Murray CJL et all, 2003). [15] Almost 37 % of under-5 population deaths are neonatal causes with 28% due to preterm births. African regions are most affected in the world(WHO, world health Report,2005) [23].This data shows that strengthening PMTCT interventions and other preventive measures will have a major impact in reducing infant mortality and improve child survival rate.

Figure1: Causes of death in Children under-5, 2000-2003

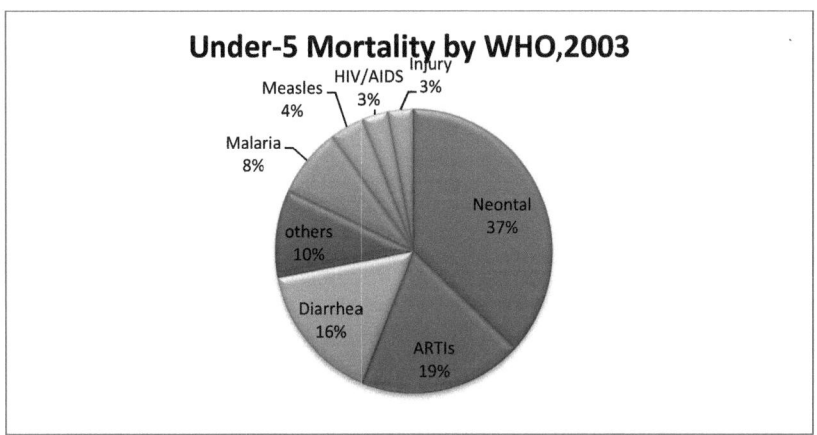

c.General objectives

The general objectives of this research paper won't be nothing else than the application of epidemiologic principles and methods to the study of HIV in neonate's population and the prevention measures. In clinical epidemiology the following outlines will be developed: from the assessment of abnormality in the general population (here the HIV-exposed neonates and infants), through the natural history, chain and mode of transmission, to the measurement of risk, treatment and prevention, a comprehensive descriptive and analytical review of PMTCT interventions and clinical presentations of HIV in this special population will be displayed to validate the daily evidence- based practices in low income countries with limited resources.

## 1. Assessing abnormality of HIV infection in Neonates

In this section, I display the context of disease abnormality in relation with HIV infection in a special population: 'the neonates".

1.1. Disease natural history

Disease natural history refers to the progression of a particular disease over time in the human body in the absence of interventions. The ultimate outcome will be recovery, disability or death. The process starts with exposure then accumulations of factors that lead to the disease manifestations and progress. Each disease has got its natural history characteristics.However; there are common steps in the development.

The next graph shows the common steps of disease natural history.

Figure 2: Natural history of disease. (CDC, 2005) [4].

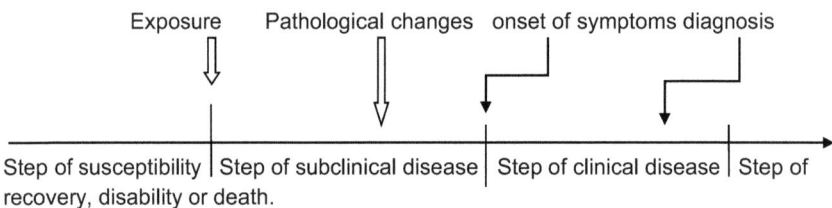

The step of subclinical disease varies from seconds (e.g. anaphylactic shock) to months (e.g. hepatitis) and decade in some diseases (e.g.cancer, HIV/AIDS).This period is called incubation period for acute infections or latent phase in chronic diseases. Although symptoms and signs of disease are unapparent during this period, more diseases can be detected whether by some laboratory investigations, radiology procedures or screening tests. It's very important to understand that screening tests should have high sensitivity and specificity to classify who has the disease and who does not among the population exposed. The advantage is that the earlier the diagnosis, the better the outcome (see chapter 2). The onset of symptoms marks the beginning of clinical stage. Most diagnosis are made during this period. Three terms are used to describe the disease progression along with the natural history of disease.

-Infectivity: This is the fraction of **exposed** people who become **infected**.

-Pathogenicity: this is the fraction of infected people who develop the **clinical disease.**

-Virulence: the fraction of people with clinical disease who develop a severe illness and may die.

Some diseases have high infectivity or pathogenicity or virulence than others.

For instance, HIV has a high infectivity, pathogenicity and virulence in neonates population. Around 30-40% of HIV exposed babies will contract the disease and half of them (50%) will die before their second birthday in absence of interventions (Newell ML et all, 2004). [17]

The natural history of HIV in neonates' population is basically following the same steps as mentioned above. The exposed period which happens in utero (5 % infections), perinatally (10-20% infections) and during breastfeeding (10-20% infections); the subclinical stage (called asymptomatic); the clinical stage (symptomatic disease, classified by WHO from mild to severe form of the disease) and the last stage which is survival or death. The immunity response which is still naive and immature, make the complexity of diagnosis and clinical futures of HIV in early life. The absolute number of CD4 cells (target cells for HIV) is normally high in neonates and can mislead the clinician. However a clinical approach for early diagnosis using clinical WHO classification or IMCI algorithm have been develop and some threshold immunity values for early treatment as well (Mark W,2010).[13]

1.2. Chain of infection

The traditional epidemiologic triad elucidate the dynamic of disease occurrence when an agent leaves its reservoir (natural habitat|) to colonise a host under some favourable environmental circumstances (see Figure 3). Benenson A.S. (as cited in Park K., 2009) defined a source of infection or reservoir as 'any person, animal, object, soil, plant or substance (or combination of these) in which an infectious agent lives and multiplies, on which its depends primarily for survival, and where it reproduces itself in such manner that it can be transmitted to a susceptible host".[18]

Figure 3:Epidemiologic triad

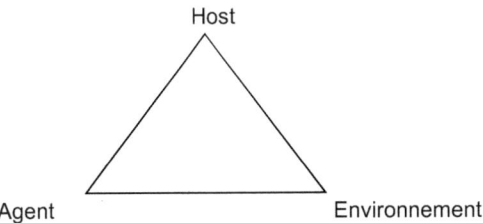

The HIV is found in a human reservoir where its replicates and cause AIDS. The virus is a RNA virus transmitted mostly sexually and vertically from the mother to the child. The chain of infection in unborn babies and neonates passes through some "portal of exit" (placenta, vaginal secretions or fluid, breast milk) to some "portal of entry" in the newborn (Immune cells, skin lacerations, gastro-intestinal tract).

1.3. Mode of transmission

After an agent exits its natural habitat, it can be transmitted to a susceptible host in many ways:

-Directly: by contact or droplet spread

-Indirectly: airborne (e.g. Tuberculosis), vector borne (e.g. malaria).

The transmission of HIV to the neonates is a vertical direct transmission of the virus from the mother to her child during pregnancy (ante partum), during labour and delivery (intrapartum) or breastfeeding (postpartum). [9] Without interventions almost 40 % of HIV-exposed infants will contract the virus and mostly 50 %of them will die before their first birthday (see figure4). The transmission occurs when the two blood circulation systems are in contact, meaning measures should be put in place during labour and delivery, time of high risk, to avoid the two circulation contact. These include reducing contact with blood serum and liquid for the labour attendant as well as avoiding any kind of intervention like episiotomy unless highly recommended.(Akani C akani,2006) [1]. The diagnosis of HIV in early stage of life is a key determinant for the reduction of vertical transmission of HIV at different levels.

Figure 4: Percentage of HIV transmission in exposed infants

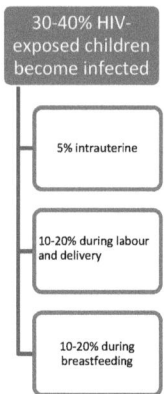

## 2. Evidence-based of PMTCT interventions

2.1. Material and methodology

For this research paper focused on PMTCT, we selected data for 3 years study from 2008 to 2010.This was a retrospective cohort study. The data included all pregnant women who attended ANC, those who were counselled and tested for HIV and those who delivered at the facility. Our indicators for the PMTCT interventions were pregnant women on HIV treatment (short course or full HAART), the number of HIV exposed babies who tested positive by DNAPCR and HIV antibody testing, the still births and those initiated on HIV prophylaxis. Patients' registers from Maternity, ANC, paediatric ward, laboratory, and ART clinic and hospital annual report were used.

2.2. Diagnostic of HIV in neonates and infants.

The gold standard of the diagnosis of HIV infection in neonates is based on the finding of the virus genomic material in the neonates' blood. The test is called "DNA PCR".

In 1989, scientists selected a polymerase chain reaction (PCR) as the major scientific innovation of the year. [7] This is the only acceptable test recommended actually for the diagnosis of HIV in children below 18 months of age though its limitations in some cases with high rate of false positive(Shah I,2004) .[19] The RNA PCR test is used only for monitoring of the virus in infected patients especially when they are on treatment. In some settings, RNA PCR is used as a confirmatory test because it has been shown somewhat more sensitive. The HIV viral culture is more accurate but very expensive for screening in routine practice. The antibody tests are not reliable for babies because they cannot distinguish between maternal and infant HIV antibodies. In medicine, the accuracy of a test is measured by its sensitivity and specificity.

In our setting, two DNA PCR test are recommended to confirm the diagnosis of HIV in exposed infants. One is done at 6 weeks or soon as after and another one at 6 months. A rapid test (HIV antibody test) is also done for all infected children at 18 months. If a child is breastfeeding, he is still at risk of HIV throughout the time of breastfeeding. A confirmatory test is performed 1 week after cessation of breastfeeding if tested negative previously.

2.2.1. Statistical testing: Sensitivity and specificity

The bottlenecks in the use of diagnostic and screening tests are to identify the proper trade-off between the people who have really the disease from those who do not have it. (Wassertheil-smoller S, 2004). [22]

Some epidemiological concepts should be understood.

-Sensitivity: the sensitivity of a test is the probability of individuals having the disease and have tested positive (true positive).

-Specificity: this is defined as the probability of individuals having the disease and have tested negative (true negative).

-Predictive value positive: This is the probability of having a disease giving a positive result.

-Predictive value negative: This is the probability of not having a disease given a negative result.

 The next 2x2 contingency table is the best epidemiologic way to summarize data for analysis/test for association. The table has two variables displayed in 2rows and 2 columns.

Table 1: Sensitivity analysis table

| Diagnostic test | True condition/Presence of the disease | | Total |
| --- | --- | --- | --- |
| | YES(+) | NO(-) | |
| Positive | a(True positive) | b(False positive) | a+b |
| Negative | c(False negative) | d(True negative) | c+d |
| Total | a+c(all diseased) | b+d(all non diseased) | a+b+c+d(total population enrolled) |

a+b=all testing positive

c+d=all testing negative

a+b+c+d=Total population

Therefore, the following formula:

-Sensitivity=$\frac{a}{a+c}$ x100     -Predictive value of a positive test=$\frac{a}{a+b}$x100

-Specificity=$\frac{d}{b+d}$ x100     -Predictive value of a negative test=$\frac{d}{c+d}$x100

-Accuracy of a test: the proportion of all tests that are correct classification

$$=\frac{a+d}{a+b+c+d}$$

Test with100% sensitivity and 100% specificity would be positive for everyone with the disease and negative for everyone without the disease. Most tests do not provide such distinction. Most of the time 2 tests, symptoms and signs are combined to improve both sensitivity and specificity of a test. (Kenneth Rothman, 2002). [10]

For instance, when using a DNA PCR for the diagnosis of HIV in exposed infant which is the gold standard test, studies has shown a low sensitivity in the first few days of life but increased in the next 2-3 weeks up to more than 90%.At 28 days, the HIV PCR has 96% sensitivity and 99 % specificity.[8] This simply means if 100 babies with disease are tested, 96 will test positive for HIV (true positive) and 4 will be missing (false positive). In the other hand, if 100 babies without the disease are tested, 99(99%) will be negative (true negative) and 1 (1%) will be missing (false negative).

2.2.2. Predictive values

The important of a diagnostic test lie on its predictive value.

-The positive predictive value of a test is the probability of a disease with a positive test.

-The negative predictive value of a test is the probability of an absence of a disease with a negative result.

Sensitivity and specificity of a test are theoretically fixed, but the predictive value depends on the sensitivity and specificity and more importantly on the prevalence of the disease (Bonita, 2006) [3]. If the disease has a low prevalence the predictive value would be very low. The opposite is also applicable.

The following table displays the data of HIV DNA PCR results in exposed infants per age groups at our institution from 2008 to 2010.

Table 2: Results of HIV DNA PCR among Exposed infant from 2008 to 2010

| Age group(months) | DNA PCR negative | DNA PCR positive | Totals |
|---|---|---|---|
| 0-3months | 27 | 1 | 28 |
| 4-6 months | 43 | 1 | 44 |
| 7-9 months | 14 | 4 | 18 |
| 10-12 months | 12 | 2 | 14 |
| 12-15 months | 4 | 0 | 4 |
| 16 and above | 0 | 1 | 1 |
| Totals | 100 | 9 | 109 |

Figure 5: HIV DNA PCR results per age category in exposed infants from 2008-2010.

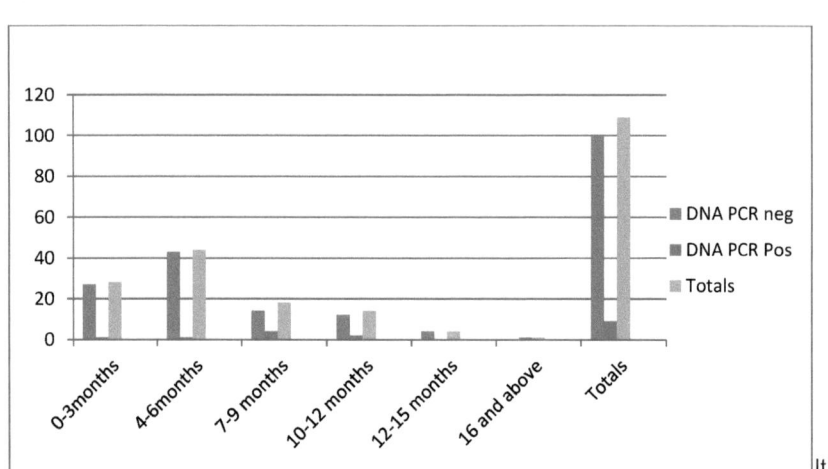

It clearly seen that the positive results are more in the age group of 6 to 9 months with 5 DNA PCR positive results(4,58%) of the total HIV exposed infants.

To test the sensitivity of the DNA PCR, we use the same data in Table 2 using a comparative method between the DNA PCR and HIV antibody test. All exposed infants were retested at 18 months using an HIV antibody kit regardless of their previous results. The statistical test is presented in table 3.

Table 3: Statistical tests of HIV DNA PCR results in HIV-exposed infant from 2008 to 2010.

| DNA PCR | HIV antibody test | | Total |
|---|---|---|---|
| | + | - | |
| Positive | 9 | 0 | 9 |
| Negative | 1 | 99 | 100 |
| Total | 10 | 99 | 109 |

The data included all DNA PCR results for both infants born at home (tested during some outreach HIV campaign activities) and at the facility who were tested during the post natal reviews at MCHC (Mother-Child health clinic).

Among the total 9 DNA PCR, only 7 were delivered at the hospital.2 were delivered at home.

-Sensitivity=$\frac{9}{10}$ x100=90%   -Predictive value of a positive test=$\frac{9}{9}$x100=100%

-Specificity=$\frac{99}{99}$ x100=100%-Predictive value of a negative test=$\frac{99}{100}$x100=99%

-The accuracy of the DNA PCR Test=108/109x100=99%.

The implication of this analysis denotes that a positive result (90%) is likely to be repeated for a confirmation of the diagnosis. And a negative result (100%) is likely to confirm that the infant has no disease and provide earlier reassurance to the clinician and the family, though another test is required if breastfeeding.This was also found in other studies (Murphy R.,Peters V.,Gill B. Et all,2004). [16]

2.3. Risk

Risk is defined as a measurement of occurrence of new cases in a population as fraction of persons at risk at a particular time.

In this review, the concept of risk is understood when considering all children born from HIV positive mothers (HIV exposed infants).

   A risk factor refers to an aspect of personal habits or environmental exposure that is associated with an increased probability of occurrence of a disease (Bonita R et all, 2006) [3].

Since risk factors are multiple and are subject to change over time, it's important to use them effectively and if possible act on them to reduce the risk of disease occurrence.

Risk factors may include obesity, hypertension, age, sex, marital status, occupation, physical activity, diet, etc

Using table 4, the risk of having a DNA PCR positive result in HIV exposed infant

Is calculated as total number of HIV exposed babies with positive results/total number of HIV exposed babies at risk at a particular time=9/113=7,9.

In epidemiology mostly a relative risk called also a hazard ratio is used to determine the risk of occurrence of an event among the exposed and non-exposed population.

## 2.3.1. Measure of relative risk

Table 4.Cumulative of PMTCT deliveries from 2008 to 2010

| PMTCT modules | frequency | Pregnancy Outcomes | frequency |
|---|---|---|---|
| Total women attended ANC | 1693 | Total who delivered at the facility | 1100(65%) |
| Total counselled and tested for HIV | 1588 (93, 7%) | Total HIV+ who delivered at the institution | 107(9.7%) |
| Total tested HIV positive | 113(7, 1%) | Total still births born from HIV+ | 7(6.5) |
| Total initiated on short course AZT from 28 weeks | 55(48, 6%) | Total HIV- exposed babies who received NVP at birth | 68(100%) |
| Total received sd NVP at onset of labour | 100(88, 5%) | Total with DNA PCR results +(confirmatory) | 8(9, 1%) |

When analysing the above data, the average of ANC attendance is good as well as the acceptance of an HIV test which is above 90%.The prevalence rate of HIV among pregnant women is 7.1%.Among those attending ANC (65%) delivered at the facility. This means the level of home deliveries still high especially in our remote setting. This is a major challenge to PMTCT scale up program. Even the transmission rate of 9,1% is lower than in other setting where it was found 16% with almost 90%PMTCT coverage.(Bancheno W.et all,2010) [2].

In epidemiology studies, a particular interest is developed to knowing what could be the risk to develop a particular disease once some folks are exposed to a particular factor. This is likelihood called relative risk: it is the ratio of two incidence rates. The rate of developing a particular condition among the people with the exposed factor divides by the rate of developing a condition among the people without the exposed factor.

The relative risk can be calculated directly using 2x2 tables in prospective studies or case control studies.

Extracting data in table 5, we can calculate the relative risk associated with still births in HIV+ pregnant women. The following 2x2 comparative table shows the frequency distribution of still births among HIV+ and HIV- pregnant women.

Table 5: Relative risk of still births among HIV+ pregnant women who delivered at the facility from 2008 to 2010.

| Maternal status | Still birth | | Total |
|---|---|---|---|
| | YES | NO | |
| HIV positive | 7(a) | 100(b) | 107 |
| HIV Negative | 15(c) | 1085(d) | 1100 |
| Total | 22 | 1185 | 1207 |

The relative risk of still births=$\frac{7/107}{15/1100}=\frac{0,0654}{0.0136}=4.88$

2.3.2. Odds ratio.

The odds ratio is closed to the risk ratio and measures the strength of the association between the risk factors and outcomes.

Odds ratio=$\frac{\text{odds of exposure in those with the condition}}{\text{odds of exposure in those without the condition}}$

Recall that odds is calculated from a probability as

Odds=$\frac{\text{Probability}}{1-\text{probability}}$ [20]

From the formula, Odds ratio will be given by

Odds ratio=OR=ad/bc

From table 5, Odds ratio=$\frac{7x1085}{15x100}=\frac{7595}{1500}=5.06$

This association is strong and means a HIV+ pregnant woman is 5 times likelihood to have a still birth than an HIV negative pregnant woman. If this association is assumed very strong, there is need to take into account the sources of confounding and biases.meaning, there is need for another study to determine if these still births among pregnant women are due to HIV virus or other causes associated.

2.3.3. Confidence interval

Last J M, in 1988 gave the formal definition of a confidence interval as: ''a range of values for a variable of interest''. [11] In our case, the measure of treatment effect] constructed so that this range has a specified probability of including the true value of the variable. The specified probability is called the confidence level, and the end points of the confidence interval are called the confidence limits'. In practice, 95% is set as the reference for the confidence interval.

The measure of a confidence interval in a 2x2 table is given by the following formula.

$$CI = OR.e^{\pm 1.96\sqrt{\frac{1}{a}+\frac{1}{b}+\frac{1}{c}+\frac{1}{d}}} \quad [22]$$

Using data in table 5, the upper 95% CI limit would be $CI = OR.e^{+1.96\sqrt{\frac{1}{7}+\frac{1}{100}+\frac{1}{15}+\frac{1}{1085}}}$

$CI = 5.06xe^{+1.96x0.47} = 12.47$

The lower 95%CI limit would be $CI = 5.06xe^{-1.96x0.47} = 2.01$

The next table displays the data for the pregnancy outcomes among the total deliveries from our system.

Table 6: Pregnancy outcomes among HIV+ and HIIV- pregnant women from 2008-2010

| Pregnant women | frequency | Received AZT From 28 weeks | Received NVP sd | Still births | Died at 36wks | HIV DNA PCR + |
|---|---|---|---|---|---|---|
| HIV+ | 107(8.8%) | 55(51.4%) | 100(95.2%) | 7(6.5%) | 2(1.8%) | 7(6.5%) |
| HIV- | 1100 | 0 | 0 | 15(1.4%) | 5(0.45%) | 0 |
| Total | 1207 | 55 | 100 | 22(1.8%) | 7(0.57%) | 7 |

In a study conducted in Botswana in 2009,Chen j. et all [5], found an overall of still births at 2.7%(0.9,4.4 95%CI) and 3.7%(0.9,15.6 95%CI) when comparing those pregnant women on full HAART and those on short course AZT respectively. Yet in our study the overall still births is at 1.8%.Chen j.et all, reported also hypertensive complications at delivery as a high risk factor for stillbirth in HIV positive than in non-reactive women with an OR=7.2(95%CI 3.8,13.7).

2.4. Prognosis

Prognosis is the prediction outcome of a disease progression. This could be recovery, disability or death. In the modern science, especially in clinical epidemiology, anticipating a disease prognosis has become a key element for successful interventions. Medical statistics should provide all necessary data when clinicians want to establish a causal inference of a disease or the failure or success for interventions. Mostly in epidemiology, prognosis is based on case fatality rate (CFR) which is the number of death due to a particular disease in a community by the total number of people with the same disease during a particular period of time.

In the next table we present some clinical features and the outcomes of the HIV exposed infant at our facility for the period under study.

Table 7: Outcomes of HIV exposed infants from 2008-2010

| Total HIV+ pregnant women who delivered at the facility | n=107 | comments |
|---|---|---|
| Total number of live births born from HIV+ women | 100(93.5%) | |
| Total number of pregnant women who started HAART during pregnancy | 13(12.1%) | According to WHO eligibility criteria[i] |
| Total number of pregnant women who received AZT from 28 weeks | 55(51.4%) | PMTCT 2008 guidelines |
| Total number of pregnant women who received Sd NVP at onset of labour | 100(93.5%) | |
| Total number of pregnant women who received AZT+3TC for 7 days after delivery | 87(81.3%) | |
| Number of babies born from HIV+ mothers who received sd NVP within 72hrs of being born | 100(100%) | |
| Number of babies who received AZT for 7 days after been born | 88(88%) | |
| Number of babies who received AZT for 28 days after been born | 129(12%) | |
| Number of babies tested HIV+ in their first year of life | 9(8.25%) | By DNA PCR |
| Number of HIV+ babies who died within their first year of life | 2(22.5%) | RR=HR=hazard ratio=4.88(see table 2.5) |

As shown in table 2.7.the CFR of HIV is 22.5% with a hazard ratio (relative risk) of 4.88.According to our report, among these 2 babies, 1 died at 6 weeks home after been discharged. The case was reported later that parents lives very far (50km) from the institution and could not afford transport to take back the child at the hospital when he became ill. The second baby developed and died at 36 weeks of severe malnutrition while he had received AZT for 28 days. Both children were breast feeding and immunization was on going.Comparitevely to a study done in South Africa (Chopra M et all, 2010) [6], the CFR of HIV exposed infant was at 8% at 36 weeks with a hazard ratio of mortality at 36 weeks of 8.9(95%CI:6.7-11.8).And for the WHO ,globally infant mortality rate due to HIV is 3%.(see figure 1).

2.5. Treatments

HIV treatment guidelines for pregnant women and their infants have been simplified and are easy to administer.Nevetheless, in resource limited settings, constraint like long distance to health facility, ignorance and high level of illiteracy in the community, lack and shortage of qualified staff, are major contributing factor to a low PMTCT coverage.

In our study, 93.5% of pregnant women received sd NVP at onset of labour and the rate of transmission was 8.25% and 89.7% survival rate. Other intervention included AZT from 28 weeks of pregnancy and onward, AZT+3TC during labour and AZT after delivery for 7 days. (See annexe 1: WHO PMTCT protocols for 2008)

In July 2010 at the international AIDS conference in Vienna, Michel Sidibé, Executive Director of UNSAIDS said:"the virtual elimination of mother to child transmission of HIV by 2015 is sacrosanct". Statement based on outcomes of a four-country African study on mothers with HIV giving birth in 2007 and 2008.Stringer EM et all, found that half of mothers(49%) do not receive Sd NVP at the time of delivery.[21]

## 3. Discussion

Evidence based medicine has emerged in mostly all clinical, laboratory and pharmacologic sciences. In our research we analysed the PMTCT intervention in the context of HIV/AIDS among the pregnant women and their exposed babies. Firstly the analysis of HIV testing used in infants showed a sensitivity of 99% and specificity roughly 100.Based on these testing results, protocols and guidelines were have been developed by the WHO. Though in some settings, the sensitivity of the DNAPCR was reported low [19], there is need to repeat the test at least at 2 occasions to confirm the diagnosis.

The evaluation of outcomes after intervention during pregnancy and after delivery showed that HIV positive pregnant women had 5 times risk (95% CI: 2.01-12.47) to have a still birth than HIV negative women with an overall still birth at 1.8%.The CFR of HIV in neonate was at 22%, with a relative risk of 4.88.Which was lower compare to other settings were the hazard ratio was reported at 8.9(95% CI: 6.7-11.8). [6]

In our study, 93.5% of pregnant women received sd NVP at onset of labour and the rate of transmission was 8.25% and 89.7% survival rate. This report is an evidence of PMTCT intervention and we believe with appropriate measures to address the challenges in low income countries the virtual elimination of paediatric transmission could be achieved.

Therapeutic protocols for the treatment of HIV in exposed and infected children are various and complex in their application. In resource limited settings, accessibility to antiretroviral drugs in the prevention of MTCT is not at 100 % as said above. There so many differences between countries and within countries. Treatment guidelines are not fully administered for several reasons:

-High level of ignorance and illiteracy among population in low resource settings.

-Long distances to health facility (e.g.50km from the village to the facility).

-High level of stigma in some communities.

-Opt out option for HIV testing.

-High rate of home delivery and challenges of taking sd NVP when not supervised.

-Inadequate and unavailability of data on the administration of ARV prophylaxis during pregnancy and labour.

-Lack and shortage of trained professionals.

-No suitable model of integration of PMTCT services in Maternal Child Health.

-Financial constraint to massive scale up of PMTCT services.

-Managerial problems relating to programmatic, communication, human resource and specialised services.


## 4. Recommendations

The virtual elimination of HIV transmission from the mother to the child by 2015 is possible if the above challenges are addressed in health care programs and plans.

-There is need of strong community involvement in health participation by massive dissemination of health information and educational materials (health promotion).

-Integration of PMTCT services in Maternal and child clinics as well as outreach programs like UCI campaigns in the community is a strong link to successful PMTCT service delivery.

-Fight stigma by involving village head men and prioritise a family -centred approach to testing and care.

-Training of qualified health professional and community health workers and traditional birth attendance in PMTCT, safe delivery and referral system.

-Employ qualified program manager focusing on health care delivery than in budget and financial management.

A study is needed to identify the particularity of these problems and address them appropriately as the complexity has gone as far as scarce of drug logistic management.

# 5 Conclusions

Evidence based medicine is an emerging discipline in all clinical and preventive medicine. In this research paper, we developed the use of epidemiology principles to demonstrate the evidence behind the importance of PMTCT interventions in a low resource setting. A total number of 1207 pregnant women had their HIV test done and had delivered at the facility. A number of 107 (8.8%) were HIV positive and 9 babies were confirmed HIV positive, bringing the transmission rate at 6.5%.

The challenges to PMTCT programs should be address urgently as we are heading to 2015 for the virtual elimination of HIV infections among the newborns. Education and community participation is a key among others for successful PMTCT interventions. Early diagnosis and care of HIV infected mothers may be a way to engage them to promote wider education messages about AIDS.

Political involvement and private-public partnership among various stake holders may be way to tackle managerial, financial and pharmaceutical challenges in the management of HIV in pregnancy and neonates.

# 6. References

1. Akani C.Akani N. (2006).HIV awareness and traditional birth practice in Niger delta area of Nigeria. *Tropical doctor, 36:208*-210.

2. Bancheno W et all. (2010).outcomes and challenges of scaling up comprehensive PMTCT services in rural Swaziland. *AIDS care 22*, no 9 p1130-1135

3. Bonita R et all. (2006). *Principles of epidemiology.*2$^{nd}$ edition .WHO press.

4. CDC (2005).*principles of epidemiology.*2$^{nd}$ edition.

5. Chen J et all. (2009).Risk factors for adverse pregnancy outcomes in Botswana.*HIV treatment bulletin.16$^{th}$* CROI, Montréal. Abstract 949.www.retroconference.org/2009

6. Chopra M et all. (2010).Survival of infants in the context of prevention of mother to child HIV transmission in South Africa. *Acta paediatrica 99*, no5 p 694-698.

7. Guyer RL, Koshland DE (1989).The molecule of the year. *Science; 246:1543*-46

8. HIV&AIDS information: babies, children and adolescents-accurate testing for babies. (n.d.) Retrieved from www.aidsmap.com

9. Institute of Medicine. (2005).Review of HIVNET 012 Perinatal HIV prevention Study. *The National academic press,* Washington D.C. www.nap.edu

10 Kenneth j.Rothman. (2002).*Epidemiology: an Introduction.* Oxford University Press Inc. p 34-35

11. Last JM. (2000) *A dictionary of epidemiology.* Oxford International Journal of Epidemiology.

12. Madon T, Hofman KJ, Kupfer L, et al. (2007) .Public health Implimentation science. *Science, 367(9509),* 449-450

13. Mark W. Kline. (2010).Paediatric HIV, *Baylor International Pediatric AIDS Initiative, November 3.*

14. Ministry Of Health, (2010) .*National Protocol Guidelines, Integrated Prevention of Mother to child transmission of HIV,* Lusaka, Zambia.

15. Murray CJL, Lopez AD, Mathers CD, Stein C. (2003).*The global burden of disease 2000 project: aims, methods and data sources. Evidence and information for policy (EIP).*WHO press, Geneva.

16. Murphy R et all. (2004).15th international AIDS conference. Bangkok, thailland.NYC *health*.

17. Newell ML, Coovadia H, Cortina-Borja M, Rollins N, Gaillard P, Dabis F; Ghent.(2004). Mortality of infected and uninfected infants born to HIV-infected mothers in Africa: a pooled analysis. *Lancet 364*:1236–43.

Doi: 10.1016/S0140-6736(04)17140-7 PMID: 1546418

18. Park K., Park's (2009).*Textbook of Preventive and Social Medicine*. 20th edition/s, Banarsidas Bhanot.India.page 90

19. Shah Ira. (2004).Diagnosis of perinatal transmission of HIV-1 infection by HIV DNA PCR, *JK Science, vol6,* No4, 187-9

20. Spiltalmic. (2006). Risk assessment 2, hospital physician. page 23-26, www.turner-white.com

21. Stringer EM et al. (2010) Coverage of Nevirapine-based services to prevent mother-to-child HIV transmission in 4 African countries. *JAMA 304* (3): 293-302

22. Wassertheil-smoller S. (2004).*Biostatistics and epidemiology: a prime for health professionals.*3rd edition, Springer.

23. WHO (2005).*World Health Report 2005, Make every mother and child count*. Report of the Director General, Geneva.

Annexe 1: WHO PMTCT Protocols for 2008

| Course | Antenatal | Intrapartum | Postnatal |
|---|---|---|---|
| When mother has received 4 weeks or more of ZDV or ART before delivery. | Mother: ZDV 300mg Twice a day starting at 28 weeks or as soon as possible thereafter | Mother: 3TC/ ZDV start dose of 2 tablets at onset of labour and 1 tablet every 12 hours until delivery. NVP 200mg single-dose at onset of labour. | Infant: NVP 2mg/kg oral suspension immediately after birth ZDV 4mg/kg twice a day for 7 days starting immediately after birth. Mother: 3TC/ ZDV 1 tablet twice a day for 7 days |
| When mother has received less than 4 weeks of ZDV or ART before delivery. | | Mother: 3TC/ ZDV start dose of 2 tablets at onset of labour and 1 tablet every 12 hours until delivery NVP 200mg single-dose at onset of labour. | Infant: NVP 2 mg/kg oral suspension immediately after birth and ZDV 4 mg/kg twice a day for 28 days. Mother 3TC/ ZDV 1 tablet twice a day for 7 days |
| When mother has received no ARV prophylaxis. | | Mother 3TC/ ZDV start dose of 2 tablets at onset of labour and 1 tablet every 12 hours until delivery. NVP 200 mg single-dose at onset of labour. | Infant: NVP 2 mg/kg as soon as possible after delivery and ZDV 4 mg/kg twice a day for 28 days. Mother 3TC/ ZDV 1 tablet twice a day for 7 days |
| .  Single dose NVP | None | Mother: Single-dose NVP 200 mg at onset of labour. | Infant: NVP 2mg/kg oral suspension immediately after birth. |

WHO ART eligibility criteria for pregnant women:CD4<350 or clinical stage 3 or 4